How to Overcome
Drug Addiction

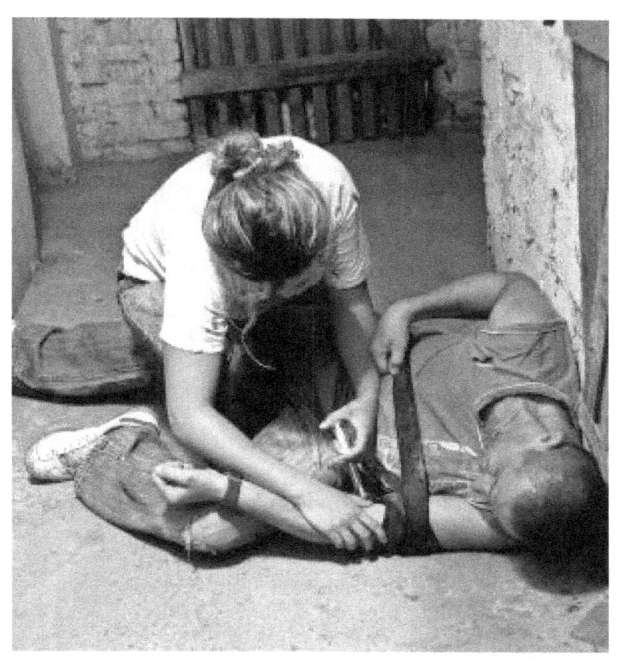

By

Colvin Nyakundi

Mendon Cottage Books

JD-Biz Publishing

All Rights Reserved.

No part of this publication may be reproduced in any form or by any means, including scanning, photocopying, or otherwise without prior written permission from JD-Biz Corp Copyright © 2014

All Images Licensed by Fotolia and 123RF.

Disclaimer

The information is this book is provided for informational purposes only. It is not intended to be used and medical advice or a substitute for proper medical treatment by a qualified health care provider. The information is believed to be accurate as presented based on research by the author.

The contents have not been evaluated by the U.S. Food and Drug Administration or any other Government or Health Organization and the contents in this book are not to be used to treat cure or prevent disease.

The author or publisher is not responsible for the use or safety of any diet, procedure or treatment mentioned in this book. The author or publisher is not responsible for errors or omissions that may exist.

Warning

The Book is for informational purposes only and before taking on any diet, treatment or medical procedure, it is recommended to consult with your primary health care provider.

Check out some of the other Health Learning Series books at Amazon.com

Health Learning Series on Amazon

Table of Contents

Introduction 4
How People Get Addicted To Drugs 5
Drug Addiction, Career and Financial Stability 11
Effects of Drug Addiction to Your Personal Life 14
How to Know if You are Addicted to Drugs 16
Commonly Abused Drugs 19
Overcoming Addiction 22
Conclusion 28
Author Bio 29
Publisher 39

How to Overcome Drug Addiction

Introduction

Drug addiction is the dependence on a drug that is psychologically or physically habit forming. In the United States alone, millions of people are addicted to one or more drugs. Overcoming addiction to drugs is one of the hardest things that a drug addict can do. You might think that the addicts don't want to stop the addiction but the truth is that the process of stopping the addiction is quite hard.

Whereas there are so many negative effects of addiction to drugs, there is no positive effect of drug abuse. Addiction to drugs has a negative impact on the addict's personal life, career, financial stability and health. With these and many more negative effects of drug addiction, you have to do everything in your power to overcome addiction to drugs.

There are several steps that you have to take if you want to overcome addiction to drugs. You can do it alone, with the help of friends and family or with the help of professionals. Start the process of overcoming addiction to drugs by reading the book "How to Overcome Drug Addiction." This book is equipped with guidelines on how to overcome drug addiction.

After reading this book, you'll know how to prevent addiction to drugs, how addiction to drugs affects your life and what you can do in order to stop addiction to drugs. Regardless of the number of years that you've been addicted to drugs, you can count on this book to help you overcome it.

You can also read this book if you want to help somebody else overcome their addiction to drugs. After reading the book, you'll also get a glimpse into some of the most addictive drugs on earth.

How People Get Addicted To Drugs

Even though all countries are trying as much as possible to get rid of illegal drugs, some people still continue to grow/manufacture and distribute these drugs. Even the legal and regulated but addictive drugs still find their way to the black market. Since it is quite difficult to stop the production, distribution and sale of addictive legal and illegal drugs, it is up to you to know how to stop addiction to drugs. Even after staying sober for several months, it is quite easy to start abusing drugs. Before learning how to overcome addiction to drugs, you need to understand how people get addicted to drugs. If you know how people get addicted to drugs, you'll know the measures to put in place so as never to get addicted to drugs.

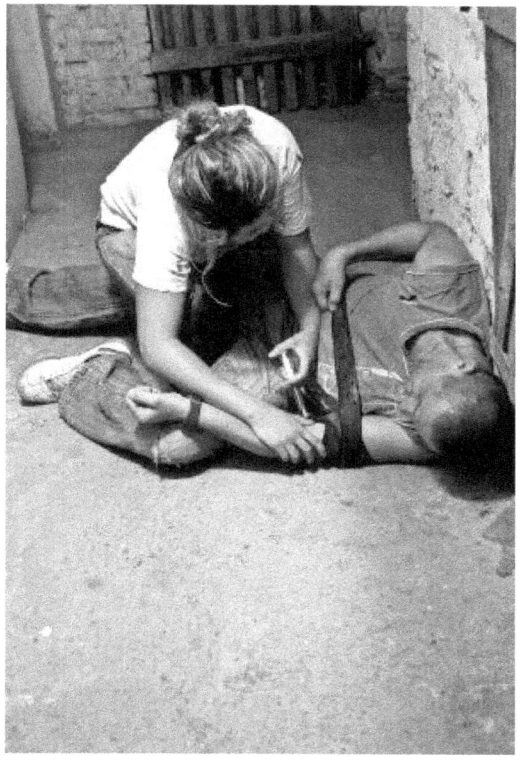

Here are some of the ways in which people get addicted to drugs:

- Hanging around drug addicts

If you have a habit of hanging around drug addicts, you're likely to start using drugs. After sometime, you'll end up being addicted to the same drugs. You also have to be very careful about who your friends are. They can trick you to start using drugs. Apart from tricking you to start abusing drugs, you can also be tempted to start using the drugs so as to feel accepted by your friends. If you want to avoid getting addicted to drugs, then you must always avoid anybody who is using illegal drugs or abusing the legal ones. However, if you notice that one of your friends is abusing drugs, don't just abandon him. Even if he/she is already addicted to the drugs, you should try as much as possible to help them overcome the addiction.

- Doing business with drug addicts

Even if you have insatiable desire to become rich, you should never do business with drug addicts. To begin with, abuse of outlawed drugs is illegal and punishable by law in all jurisdictions around the world. By simply doing business with a drug addict, you'll be exposing yourself to lawsuits. Your drug abusing business partners can also tempt you to start abusing drugs. On top of that, you can easily get tempted to start selling the drugs that your business partners are addicted to. If you want to avoid getting addiction to drugs, you must avoid doing business with drug addicts at all costs.

- Selling, transporting or dealing in drugs

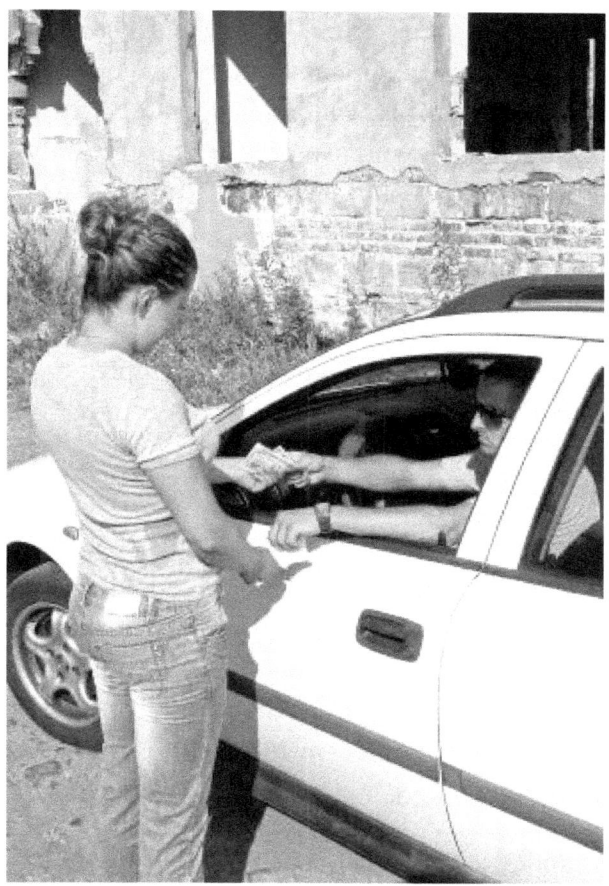

You can also get addicted to drugs if you transport, sell or distribute the drugs. Addiction to drugs is a gradual process that may take several months or even years. When selling drugs, some of your clients may want proof that you're selling a high quality product. By demanding the proof, you'll be forced to use the drugs, just to prove that they are harmless and high quality. In the long run, you'll be the one who's addicted to the drugs. If you're keen on avoiding addiction to drugs, you should never transport, sell or deal in the illegal drugs.

- Curiosity

It is quite unfortunate that some people are curious about everything in life. Such people always want to experience all events and taste everything that they come across. If you're one of those people, you should never be curious to know how drugs taste or the effect they'll have on you. Regardless of how tempted you are to try a given drug, do everything you can to avoid tasting it. This is the only way you can avoid getting addicted to that drug.

- Visiting drug dens

You can also get addicted to drugs if you have a habit of visiting drug dens. When visiting such places, you can be tempted to try the drugs just to know how the other drug users feel. After some time, you'll end up being addicted to the drugs being sold there.

- Being too idle

A wise man once said that an idle mind is the devils workshop. When you have nothing to do, your mind will wander of and start thinking of using drugs. You'll start using drugs as a way of killing the boredom. In the long run, you'll be addicted to the drug that initially helped you kill the boredom. If you're keen on avoiding addiction to drugs, you need to find something to always keep you busy.

- Stress and disappointment in life

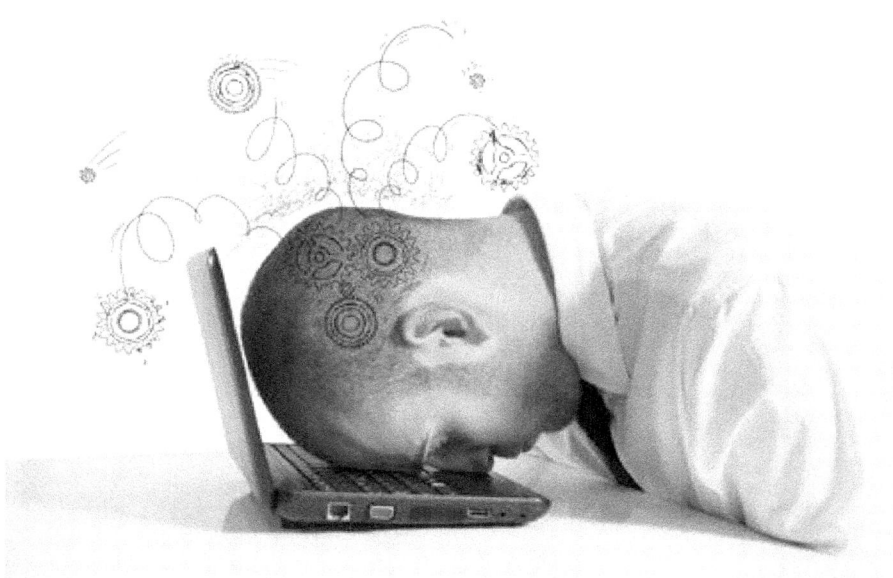

Some people resort to using drugs due to disappointments in life and stressful circumstances. You can be tempted to start using drugs as a way of coping with a stressful lifestyle. If you've been too stressed lately, then you need to take some time off and relax. You should also learn to let go of the past and forget about all the disappointments in your life.

- Low self esteem

Low self esteem is also one of the factors that can lead somebody towards drug addiction. People with low self esteem resort to using drugs as a way of making themselves feel better. You need to work on your self esteem if you want to avoid getting addicted to drugs.

- Overdose of prescription drugs

Even though prescription drugs such as morphine are manufactured for medicinal purposes only, you can easily get addicted to them if you're not too careful. Even if you feel excessive pain, you should never take an overdose of drugs prescribed by a qualified medical practitioner. Drug overdose may lead to addiction.

Drug Addiction, Career and Financial Stability

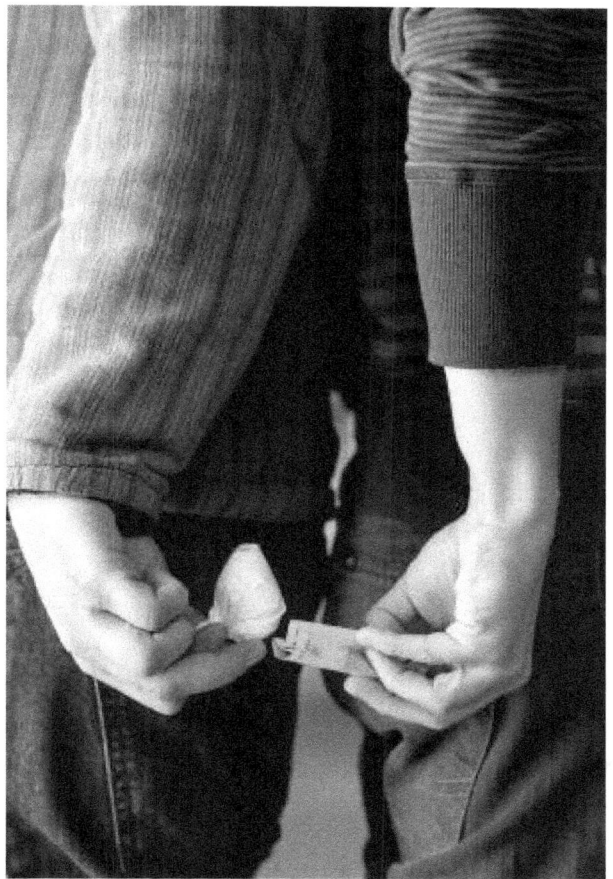

Addiction to drugs will have a huge negative impact on your career and financial status. To begin with, both the legal and illegal addictive drugs are quite expensive. This explains why it is almost impossible to find a wealthy drug addict. When addicted to drugs, you'll be spending a huge portion of your earnings on the drugs. Some drug addicts even go to the extent of buying drugs instead of buying food. With addiction, you can also be tempted to sell your investments or assets just to go buy drugs. If you ever want to become a wealthy person, you must avoid addiction to drugs at all costs.

Addiction to drugs may also lead to petty theft. Drug addicts are always willing to do anything as long as they get the money to buy drugs. A drug addict is therefore ready to steal petty stuff from his/her neighbor or colleague. Apart from petty theft, addiction to drugs can also breed hardcore criminals. This is because drug addicts don't care about what happens to them and hence they can do anything to get easy money. This therefore means that you can easily land in jail if you are a drug addict. The only way you can avoid incarceration is by avoiding addiction to drugs and hence avoiding petty and hardcore crimes.

Drug addicts also find it quite difficult to keep track of their finances. They buy stuff in bulk and without a sound budgetary plan. It is therefore almost impossible for drug addicts to manage their finances properly and hence they tend to remain poor forever. If you want financial independence, you must try as much as possible never to get addicted to any drug.

You should never rely on a drug addict to make a business decision on your behalf. This is because drug addicts have a tendency of making bad business decisions. When addicted to drugs, your judgment will be highly impaired. This means that your analytical skills will be hampered and hence you can easily make a bad choice when required to do so.

When doing business while high on drugs, you can be swindled by conmen or even your business partners. If you are the boss, you will find it quite hard to supervise your juniors when high on drugs. Your employees might steal from you without your knowledge. The only way you can make maximal profits is by ensuring that nobody ever steals from you. You should therefore avoid drug abuse if you're keen on maximizing your profits.

Addiction to drugs will also affect your level of concentration while at work. When using drugs, you're likely to lose concentration. You'll find it quite hard to meet deadlines or do a high quality job. This means that you will never be promoted. You can also get fired quite easily if you don't stop using drugs.

Effects of Drug Addiction to Your Personal Life

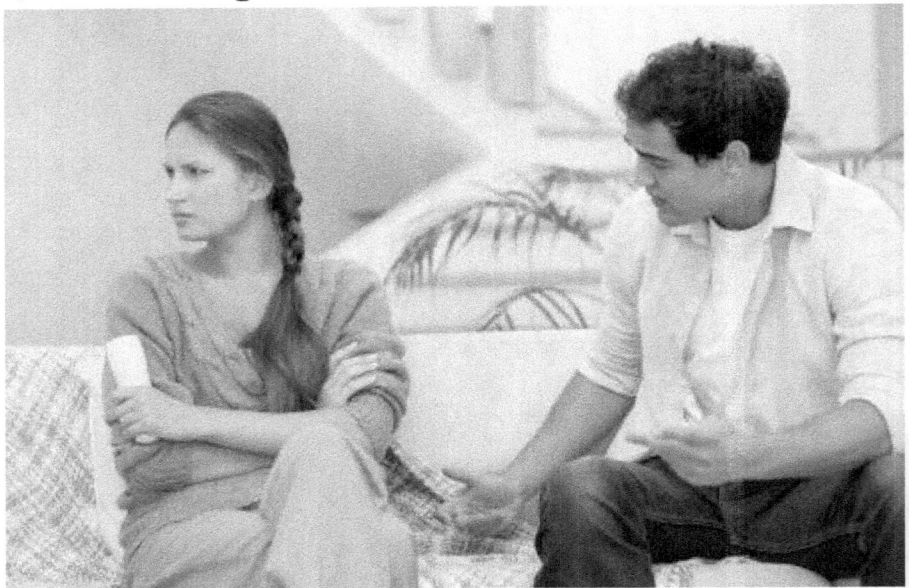

On top of affecting your career and financial status, addiction to drugs will have a negative effect on your personal life. You relationship with your parents, peers, colleagues, friends, spouse and children will be highly affected if you abuse drugs. Addiction to drugs will also affect your relationship with your bosses. When running for public office, you'll find it very difficult to convince the electorate to vote for you if you're a drug addict. Regardless of your current occupation or status in the society, you should avoid addiction to drugs at all costs.

Drug addicts find it very difficult to maintain a long term romantic relationship with anybody. They spend more time in drug dens than with their lovers. They also waste a lot of time looking for money to go buy drugs. They therefore never find quality time to spend with their lovers, children or friends.

Addicts also tend to be physically and psychologically abusive to their children, spouses and friends. This means that your kids, spouse and friends will start avoiding you if you're always high on drugs.

The only way you can have a long term relationship with them is by avoiding drug abuse at all costs.

When addicted to drugs, it will be very difficult to fend for or take care of your family. Apart from failing to provide the financial support to your family, you won't be there to provide mental support. You're also likely to forget important events in your life including your spouse's and children's birthdays. This means that you'll have a strenuous relationship with them.

If you are a drug addict, you'll never be respected or taken seriously by your peers, friends, colleagues or spouse. How do you expect other people to respect you or take you seriously if you're always high on drugs? You have to earn their respect by avoiding abuse of drugs.

Addiction to drugs will also have a negative impact on your health. Abuse of drugs generally leads to poor health. When addicted to drugs, your body will be weak and hence you're likely to fall ill frequently.

Some drugs affect your body immune system. This means that you'll be prone to so many diseases. If you're a drug addict, you'll spend money treating ailments that you could have avoided by simply avoiding addiction to drugs. Diseases such as liver cirrhosis and lung cancer can be prevented by avoiding abuse of alcohol and tobacco respectively.

Drug abuse is also likely to reduce your lifespan by a couple of years. If you're keen on living a long and healthy lifestyle, you should try as much as possible to avoid getting addicted to drugs. On top of affecting your health, your family's health will also be affected by your drug addiction. Drug addicts tend to be generally dirty and unhygienic. This means that you can easily acquire waterborne diseases.

How to Know if You are Addicted to Drugs

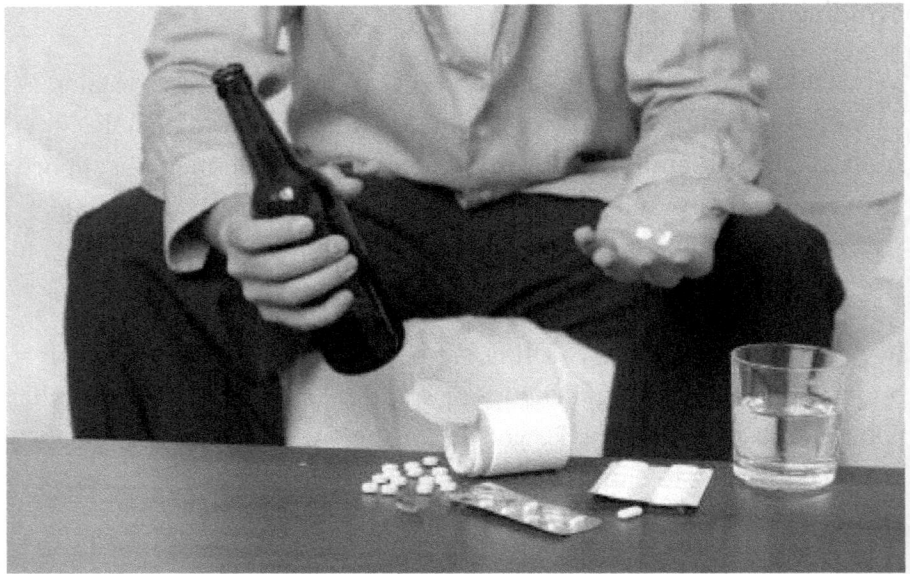

Addiction to drugs is not something that you can ever be proud of. Actually, you might be addicted to drugs but you have no idea that you're an addict. If you've been frequently using a given (legal or illegal) drug, you can know if you're addicted to it by answering the following questions.

Have you unsuccessfully tried to stop using the drug? When addicted to a given drug, it is quite difficult to stop using it. Even if you try forcing yourself to stop using the drug, it is still difficult to completely stop using it. You're therefore highly likely to be addicted to the drug if you've tried unsuccessfully to stop using the drug.

Do you experience any changes when you don't use the drug(s) as you normally do? You are likely to experience withdrawal symptoms once you stop using drugs that you're addicted to. For instance, if you're addicted to tobacco, you can experience a headache when you stay for a long period of time without smoking a cigarette. If you're experiencing withdrawal symptoms, then that implies that you are addicted to the drug.

Have you ever engaged in risky behavior while under the influence of the drug? One common thing about drug addicts is that they normally don't think straight or care about themselves or other people. Therefore, they're highly likely to engage in activities that endanger their lives or other people's lives. For instance, you can be tempted to drive your car recklessly when under the influence of alcohol than when sober. Therefore, if you notice that of late you've been engaging in risky activities after using a given drug, then you might be addicted to it.

Have you ever neglected your duties and responsibilities while under the influence of the drug? Drug addicts are normally so dependent on the drug to the extent that they'd rather use the drug than do something useful. They therefore tend to neglect their responsibilities and duties while at the same time spending more time in drug dens. If you've neglected your responsibilities on several occasions while high on a given drug, then you might be addicted to that drug.

How many times have you ever been arrested while high on the drug? A normal person will quit using a given drug if he/she is ever arrested while using it. On the other hand, a drug addict will find it quite hard to stop using the drug even after being arrested several times. If you've been arrested more than once while high on a given drug, then you might be addicted to the drug.

Do you still spend time with your family and friends? Addiction to drugs has a psychological effect on the addicts. In other words, the addict's attitude, values, and general mindset is completely changed. You could therefore be addicted to drugs if you no longer enjoy spending time with your family and friends or if you don't enjoy your hobbies as much as you used to enjoy in the past.

Other behavioral symptoms that distinguish drug addicts include self isolation from other people, erratic behavior, mood swings, unusual hyperactivity, giddiness, irritability, anxiety, paranoia, agitation, excessive secrecy, frequent fights and accidents, need for extra money, lack of accountability to anybody and changes in personal hygiene levels.

Apart from the behavioral changes, there are several physiological changes that you'll experience after you start abusing a given drug. The severity of the changes will depend on the level to which you're addicted and the quantity of drugs you are consuming. The nature of physiological change will be dependent on the type of drug you're addicted to.

Physiological symptoms of drug abuse include unusual or bad body odor, frequent tremors, excessive weight loss or gain, lack or excessive appetite, bloodshot eyes, changes in size of the pupil, slurred speech, changes in sleep patterns and abnormal body coordination.

Commonly Abused Drugs

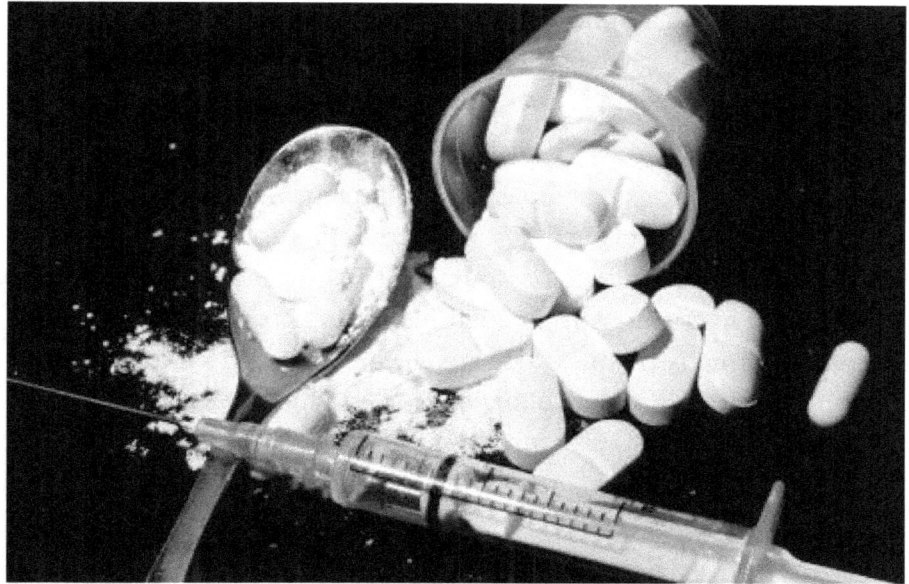

Throughout the world, there are countless legal and illegal addictive drugs in circulation. Some drugs are more common in some areas than other drugs. For instance, cocaine is more common in Central and South America than in other parts of the world. Here are some of the drugs that are widely abused in the world:

- Heroin

Heroin is a highly addictive drug that has been in circulation since time immemorial. This drug is illegalized in all jurisdictions around the world. Some of the symptoms of addiction to heroin include twitching, vomiting, abnormal sleeping patterns, contracted pupils that are not responsive to light, sweating, loss of appetite and coughing.

- Marijuana

Marijuana or cannabis is also one of the addictive drugs that are highly circulated around the world. Even though the drug is highly abused, it is also used for medicinal purposes. There are several countries and states where this drug is sold legally. When abused, the drug can result in the following symptoms: hyperactivity, weight gain or loss, glassy and red eyes and loss of interest.

- Depressants

Depressants are drugs that are used to calm a person and reduce excitability. They're also popularly referred to as sedatives. They include but are not limited to valium, GHB and xanax. If used according to instructions from qualified medical practitioners, these drugs are normally harmless. However, the following symptoms are exhibited by people addicted to depressants: clumsiness, contracted pupils, poor judgment, difficulty concentrating, slurred speech and sleepiness.

- Hallucinogens

Hallucinogens are drugs used to induce altered sensory experiences or hallucinations in patients. They include LSD and PCP. Even though these drugs are legally used for medical purposes, they still find their way into the black market and are widely abused by some addicts. Symptoms associated with hallucinogens include but are not limited to confusion, hallucinations, dilated pupils, mood swings, aggression and detachment from other people.

- Stimulants

A stimulant is any drug that temporarily quickens some vital process in a human body. For instance it could induce sleep instantly. Drugs categorized as stimulants include cocaine, crystal methamphetamine and amphetamines. These drugs are very addictive. Some of the symptoms that characterize the abuse of stimulants include euphoria, dilated pupils, abnormal sleeping patterns, weight loss, dry mouth and nose, lack of appetite, irritability and anxiety.

- Inhalants

Inhalants are drugs ingested through the nose or mouth. They include glues, aerosols and vapors. Even though these drugs are not very popular among drug addicts, they are quite addictive. Some of the symptoms that characterize addiction to inhalants include drowsiness, poor muscle control, anxiety, rashes around the nose and mouth, discharges from the nose, watery eyes, impaired vision and irritability.

Overcoming Addiction

Now that you know how people get addicted to drugs and how drugs affect your lifestyle, it will be easy to know how to overcome addiction to drugs. The first step involves acknowledging that you have a problem and that you need help. There is absolutely no way that you can overcome addiction to drugs if you still think that you're not addicted to the drugs.

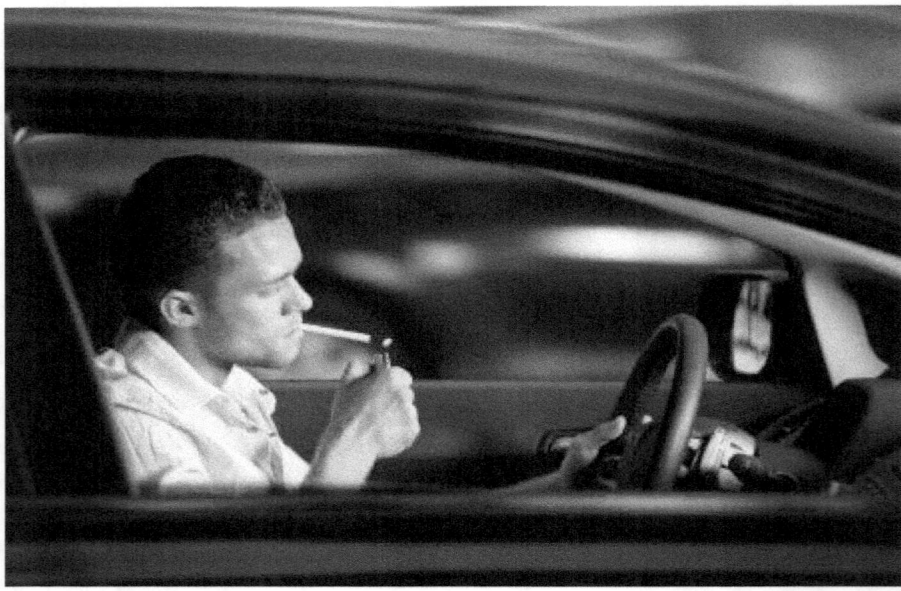

After acknowledging that you have a drug addiction problem that needs to be addressed immediately, you should change your lifestyle and daily routine. In most cases, addicts abuse drugs while doing something else. For instance, a cigarette addict will be driving while at the same time smoking the cigarette. On the other hand, an alcoholic could have a habit of drinking daily in the evenings. You can start driving your car in the company of a colleague who doesn't smoke. This way you'll be forced not to smoke so that the colleague isn't affected. You can also find something to keep you busy during the evenings so that you're not attempted to start drinking. By simply changing your routine, you can get rid of your drug addiction problem.

You also have to avoid all drug addicts even if they're your friends. By simply hanging around people who abuse drugs, you'll be tempted to start using the same drugs after staying sober for some time. Instead of hanging around drug addicts, you should make new friends who don't use the drugs. This way you'll find a way to emulate them and hence stop abusing drugs.

Some people abuse drugs because it is quite easy to access the drugs. For example, you could be addicted to alcohol simply because you stock them in your home. It is also possible that you're addicted to heroin, cocaine or methamphetamine because you have unlimited access to people selling such drugs. So as to stop your addiction, make sure that you can't access the drugs. Start by getting rid of all the stock that you've piled in your home. While getting rid of the drugs in your home, don't give them away to other drug addicts or sell them. If possible, destroy the drugs completely.

After getting rid of all the drugs, you need to delete all drug dealers' contact information. There is no way you can stop abusing drugs if you still have the contact details of drug dealers. With the contact information, you'll be tempted to call them as soon as you have a craving for the drugs. You can also try convincing the drug peddlers to stop dealing in drugs.

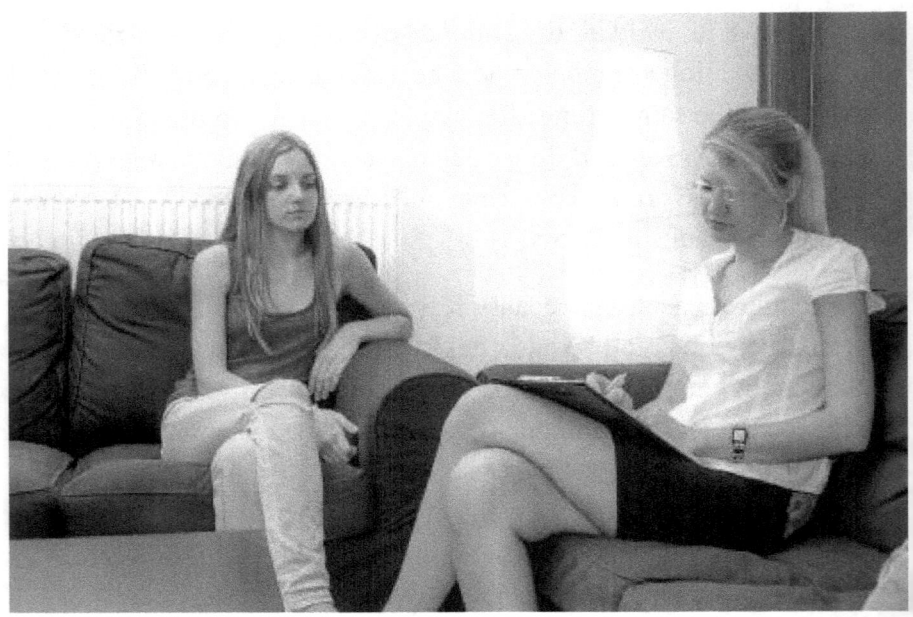

There are several predisposing factors that make people abuse drugs. Some people abuse drugs when they feel stressed or depressed. Loneliness and isolation from other people can also lead to drug abuse. It is also possible to start abusing drugs as a result of peer pressure. So as to get rid of your drug addiction problems, you have to avoid all these predisposing factors. If for example you're tempted to use drugs when depressed, you can talk to a psychotherapist to help you deal with depression. You should also make new friends and interact with as many people as possible so as not to be lonely.

You can also overcome addiction to drugs by talking to friends, family and anybody else who cares about you. Nobody who cares for you will ever want to see you addicted to drugs. This means that they'll be there to give you guidance and financial support when you're trying to stop using drugs. By simply opening up to them and sharing your problems, you can overcome the addiction.

Apart from talking to the people that care about you, try to interact with people who used to be addicts but are now not addicted to any drug. Ask them what they did to overcome the addiction. You can also emulate their lifestyles and see if you can be able to overcome your addiction to drugs.

You can also overcome addiction to drugs by use of recommended medication or alternatives to the drugs. For example, you can decide to smoke an electronic cigarette instead of an actual one with traces of tobacco. This way, you'll feel like you're smoking something but you won't be consuming tobacco which is harmful to your health. Eventually, you'll overcome the addiction to drugs as you won't have the craving for tobacco.

Whenever you have a craving for a given drug, try thinking of all the bad things that have happened to you since you started using the drug. Imagine of all the assets that you used to own before you sold them to go buy drugs. Think of how your family and personal life has been negatively affected by your addiction. You can also think of how you've stagnated in your career since you started using the drugs. By simply thinking of all the negative effects of your drug addiction problem, you will have the strength and courage to stop using the drugs. This means that you will eventually overcome the drug addiction.

You stand to gain a lot by quitting drug abuse. To begin with, you will save a lot of money since most addictive drugs are quite expensive. Within a few months of stopping drug abuse, you will have enough money to invest in your future. Your productivity while at work or home will also improve significantly once you stop abusing drugs. You will therefore get a promotion and have a better relationship with your spouse. If you want to overcome your drug addiction problem, try thinking of all these and many more benefits that you stand to gain.

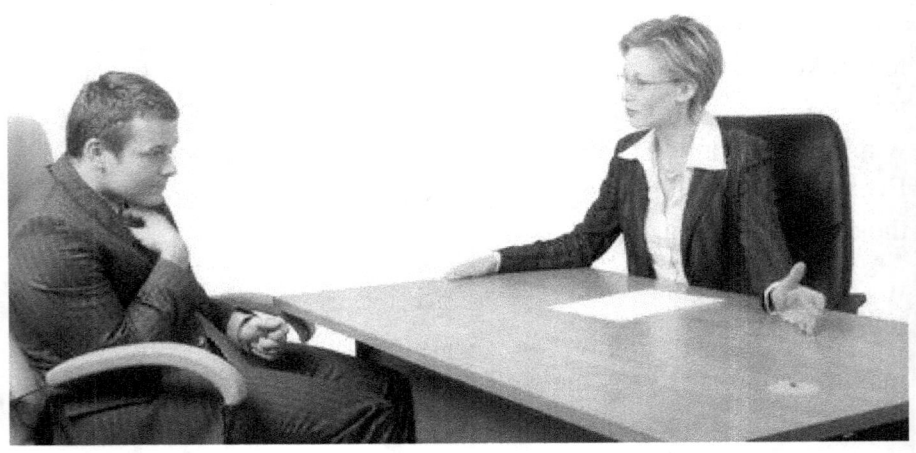

To overcome drug addiction, you should be accountable to someone in your life including your spouse, children, parents or boss. Being accountable basically means being answerable to them. If you're accountable to someone, you will feel obliged not to use any drug as you will have to explain why you decided to take the drugs. You should be accountable to someone who is in a position to punish or castigate you whenever you abuse the drug(s). This way you can stop using the drugs out of fear that you'll be punished if you're caught high on the drug.

Identifying a mentor can also help you stop drug addiction. A mentor is a trusted guide who can give you sound advice whenever you seek their assistance. He/she should be somebody who is highly respected in the society; someone to look up to. The mentor should also be morally upright and not controversial in any way. Your mentor should be someone you can access at any time of the day. It is also very important that the mentor shouldn't be addicted to any drug. Once you've identified a mentor, you should try to emulate him/her. This way you can stop abusing drugs and hence overcome addiction.

If you've unsuccessfully tried to quite drug addiction, then you need to enroll in a drug rehabilitation program. There are so many drug rehabilitation centers in the United States as well as in all the other countries. Identify a center with high integrity standards and that has helped several people overcome drug addiction. The most important thing is to make sure that you do everything you're told by instructors in a drug rehabilitation center. After a few weeks or months (depending on your level of addiction) you will get out of the rehabilitation center without a craving for the drugs.

When trying to overcome addiction to drugs, you should never stop using the drugs instantly. This is because you will suffer from withdrawal syndromes. There have been several reported deaths as a result of instant drug withdrawal. It is always advisable that you follow the step by step guidelines on how to overcome drug addiction.

Conclusion

Drug addiction is a universal problem that affects everybody in the society regardless of their status, career or wealth. Even though you might not be a drug addict, you will be affected by drug addicts in one way or another. It is therefore your responsibility to make sure that those close to you are not addicted to drugs. If you have just overcome drug addiction, then you must do everything in your power to ensure that you won't become a drug addict again.

Apart from dealing with addiction to drugs, it is also important to prevent the addiction beforehand. This is because overcoming addiction to drugs is quite expensive and may drain your finances. So as to understand how much money you need in order to overcome drug addiction, try enquiring how much it costs to enroll in a drug rehabilitation center.

To prevent addition to drugs, you should do everything in your power to stop the production/manufacture, distribution and sale of illegal drugs. However, if you are already addicted to drugs, you can overcome the addiction by implementing the ideas discussed in this book. You can also use these ideas to help a friend, colleague or family member overcome his/her addiction to drugs.

Good luck overcoming or helping someone overcome their addiction to drugs!!!

Author Bio

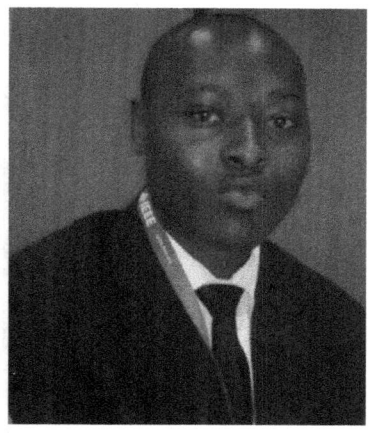

Colvin Tonya Nyakundi is a freelance writer and co-author of 'How to Overcome Drug Addiction". Apart from that book, he has a portfolio of several other publications accumulated in the more than two years that he has been freelancing through www.odesk.com.

He has authored several personal relationships, construction and real estate, lifestyle and travel and holiday guide publications. Other books that he has co-authored include 'How to Survive in the Woods', 'How to Start Making Money Online', 'How to Survive in a Desert', 'How to Improve Your Communication Skills,' 'Construction Guide for New Investors in Real Estate,' 'How to Make Your Backyard a Magnificent Venue for Hosting Events', 'How to Identify the Perfect Holiday Destination', 'How Your Favorite Meal Could be Killing You Slowly', 'How to Get a Promotion at Work' and 'How to Prepare and Survive in a Foreign Country.' You can get in touch with him through his official Facebook account, tonyanc@facebook.com.

Check out some of the other JD-Biz Publishing books

Gardening Series on Amazon

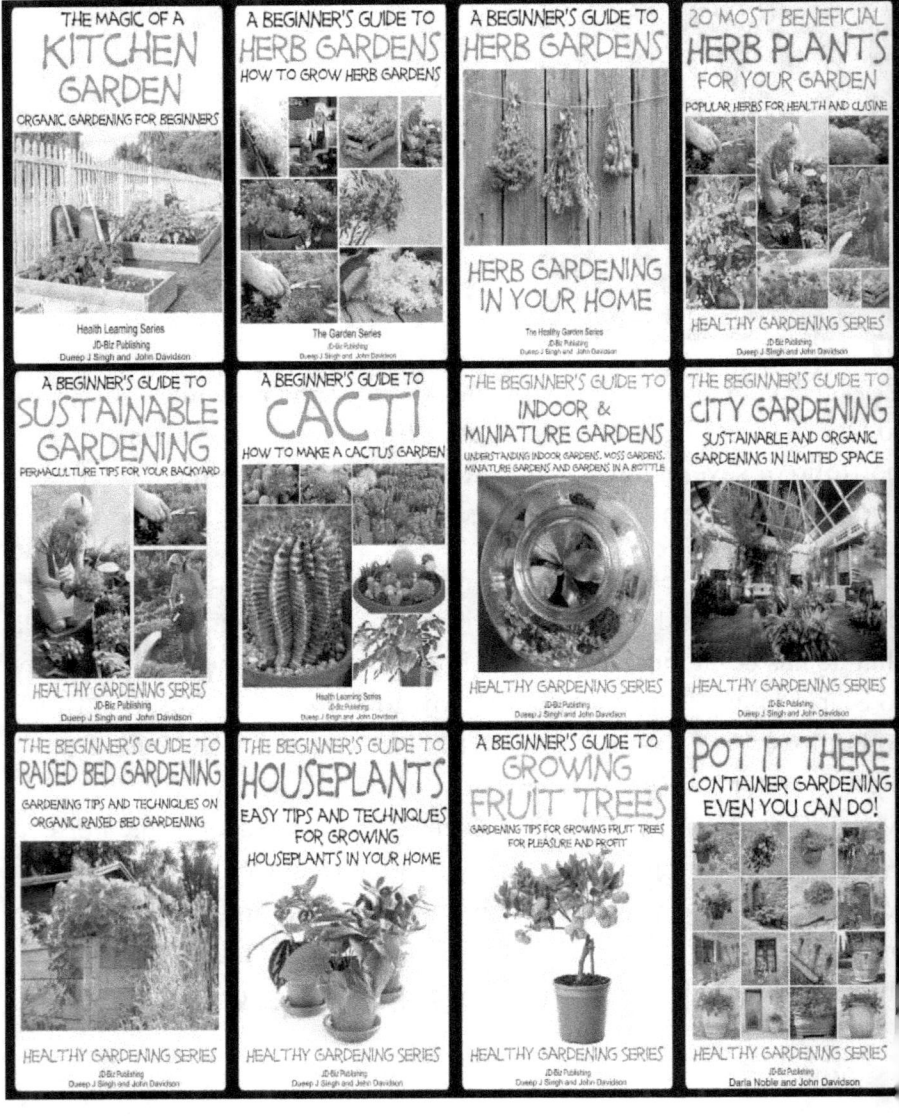

Health Learning Series

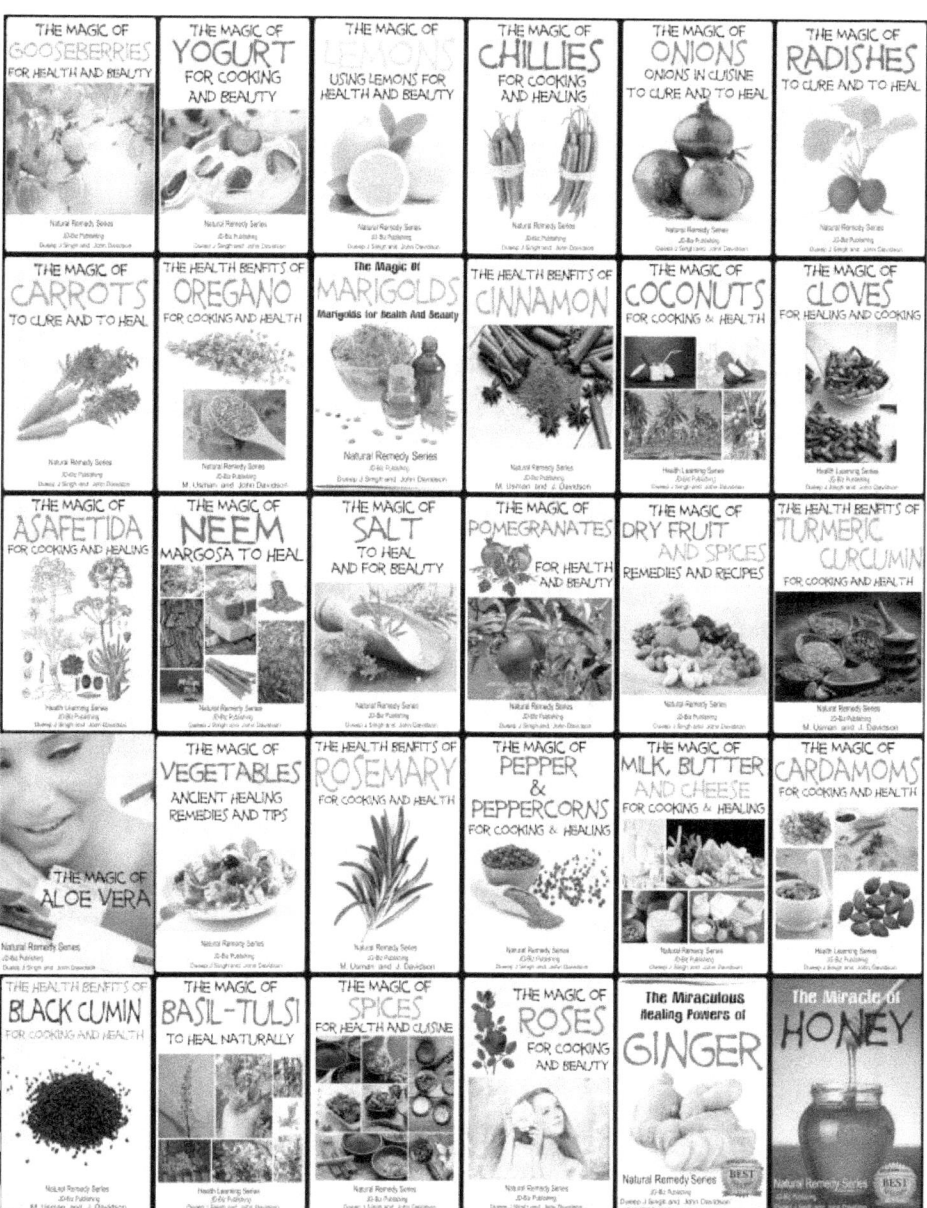

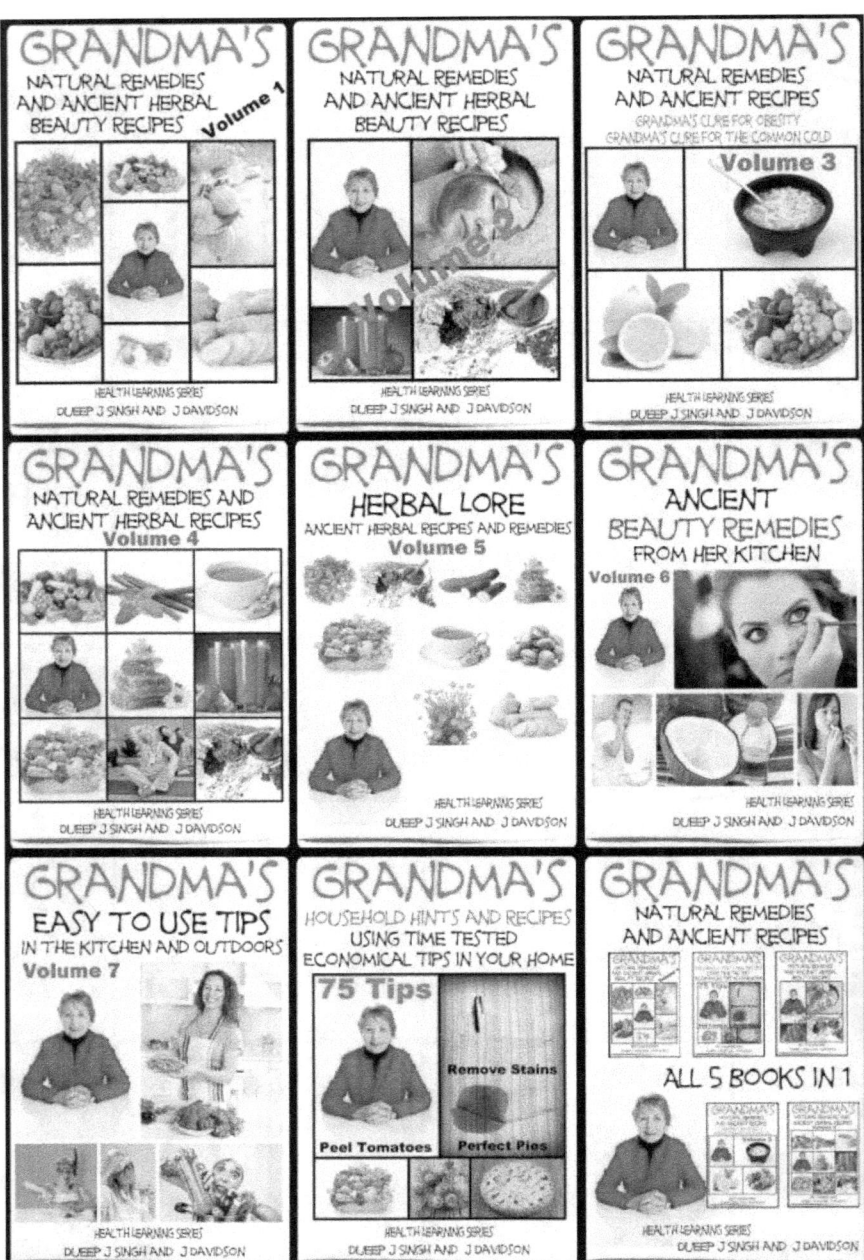

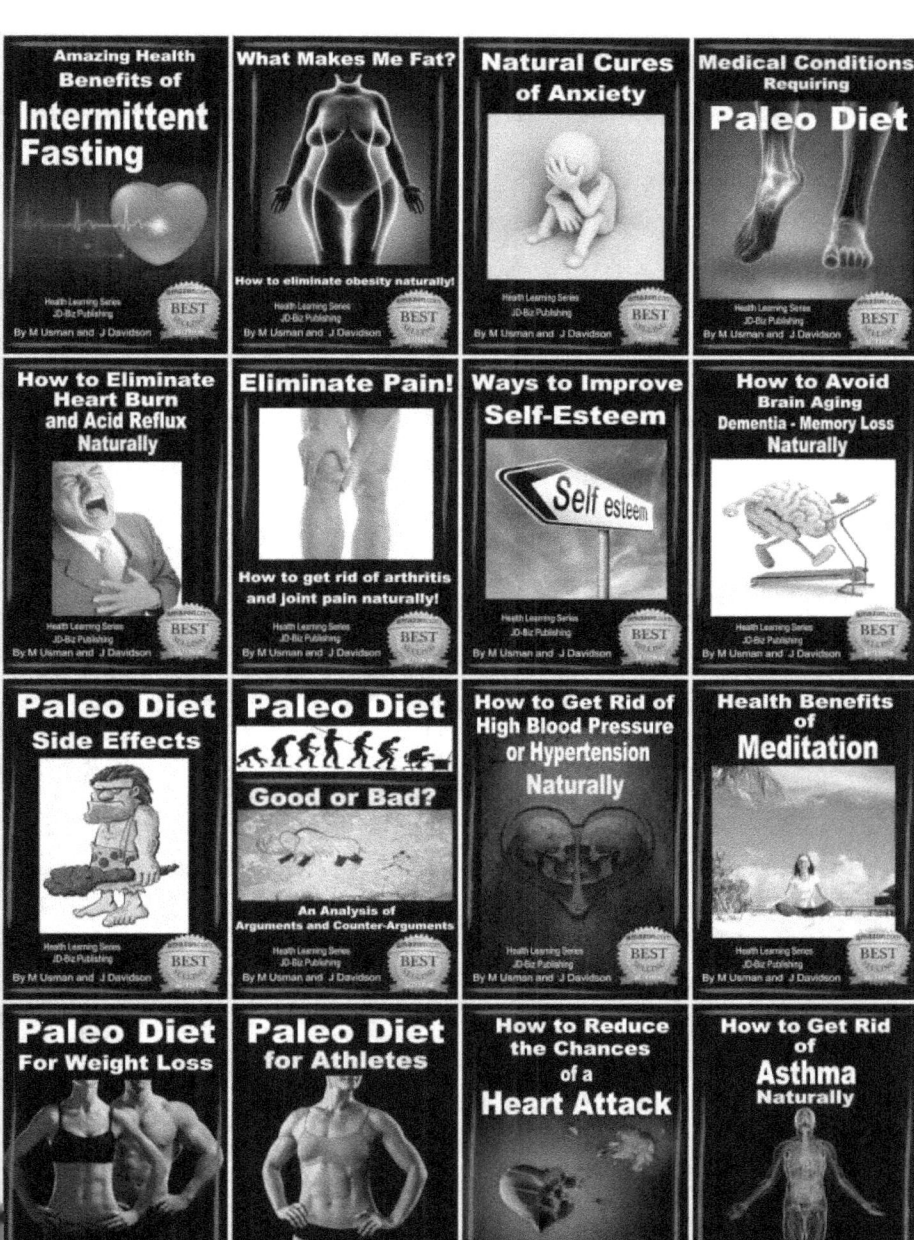

Amazing Animal Book Series

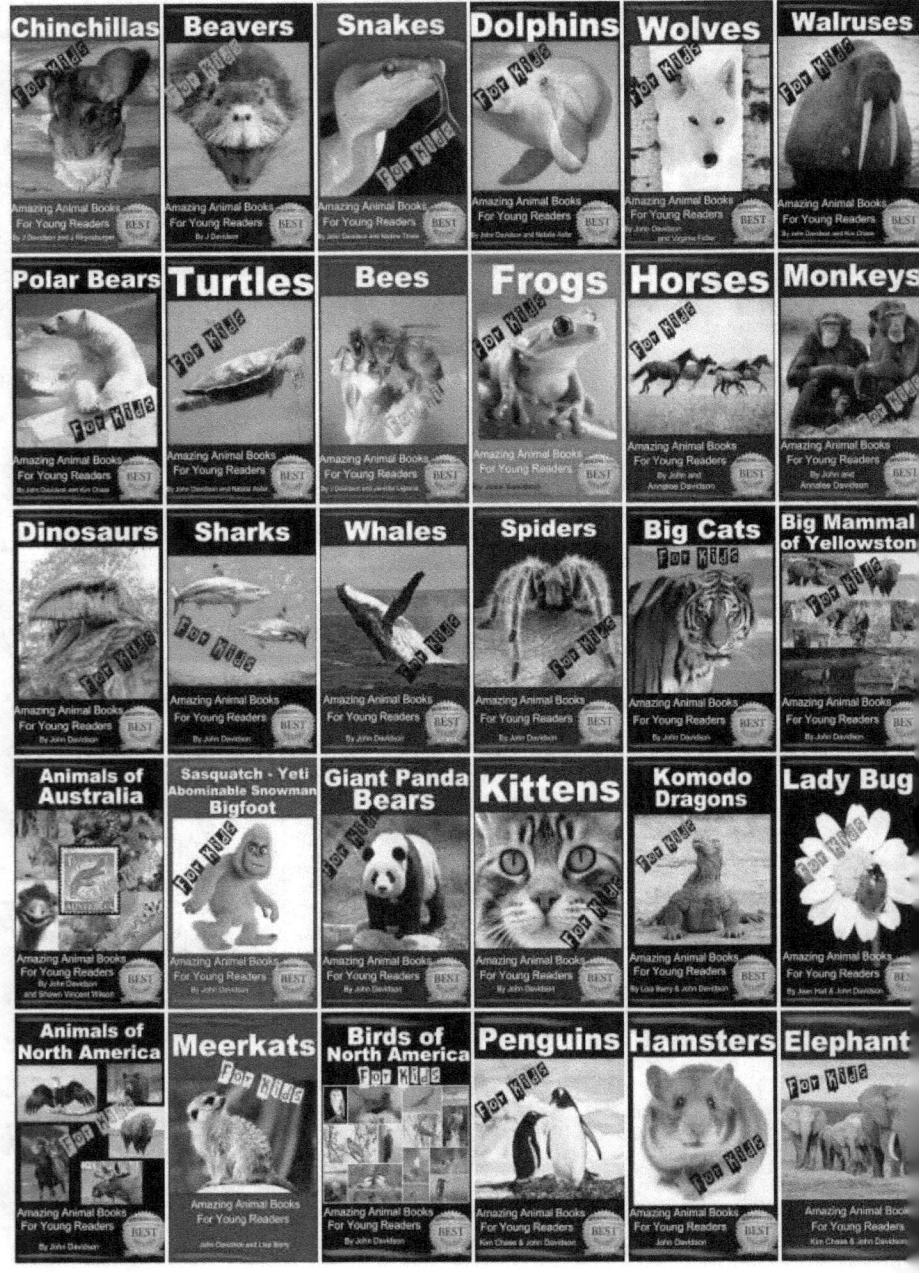

Learn To Draw Series

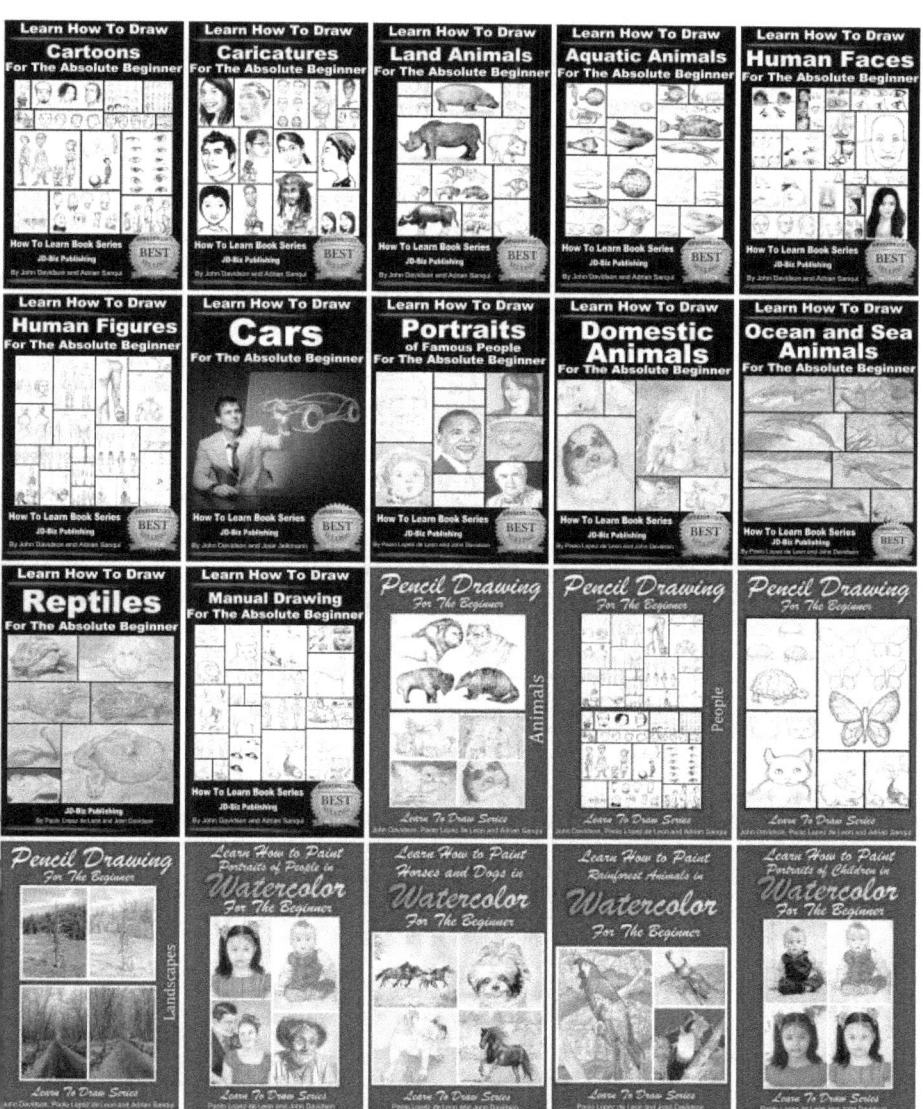

How to Build and Plan Books

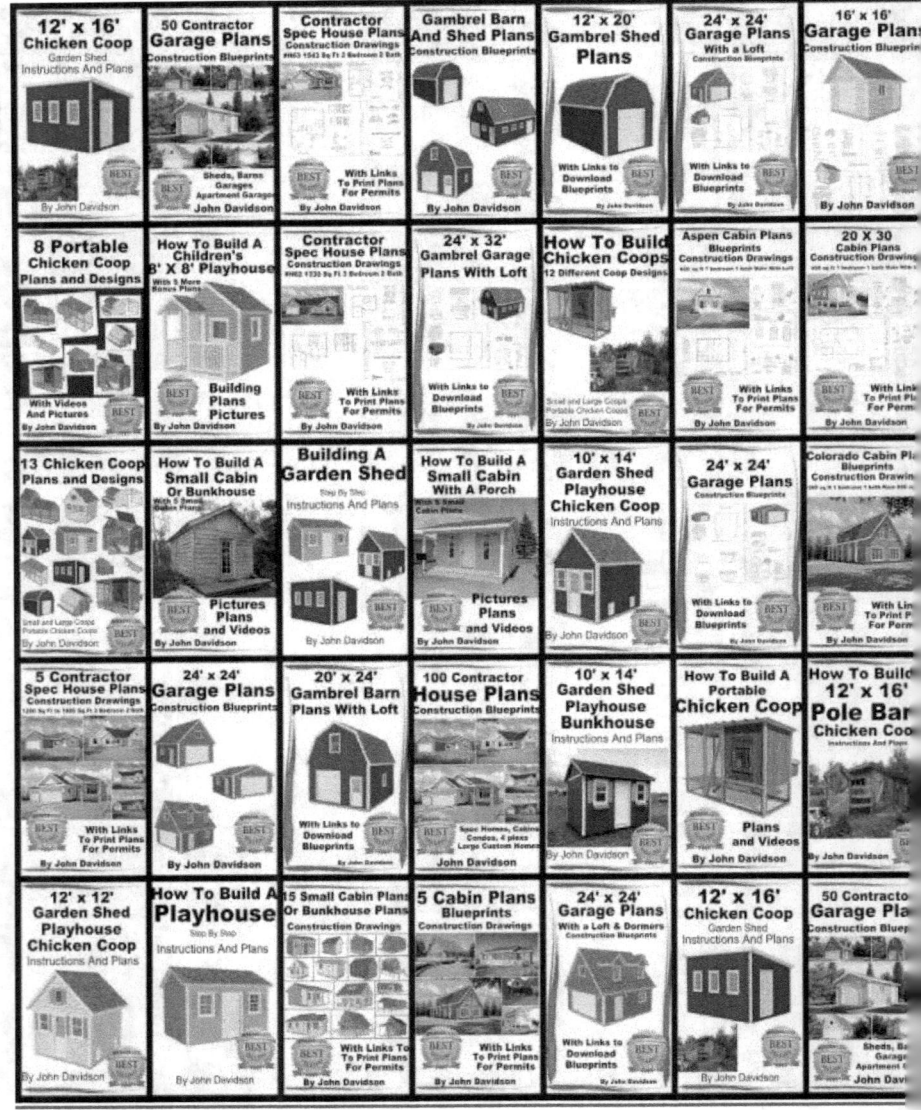

Entrepreneur Book Series

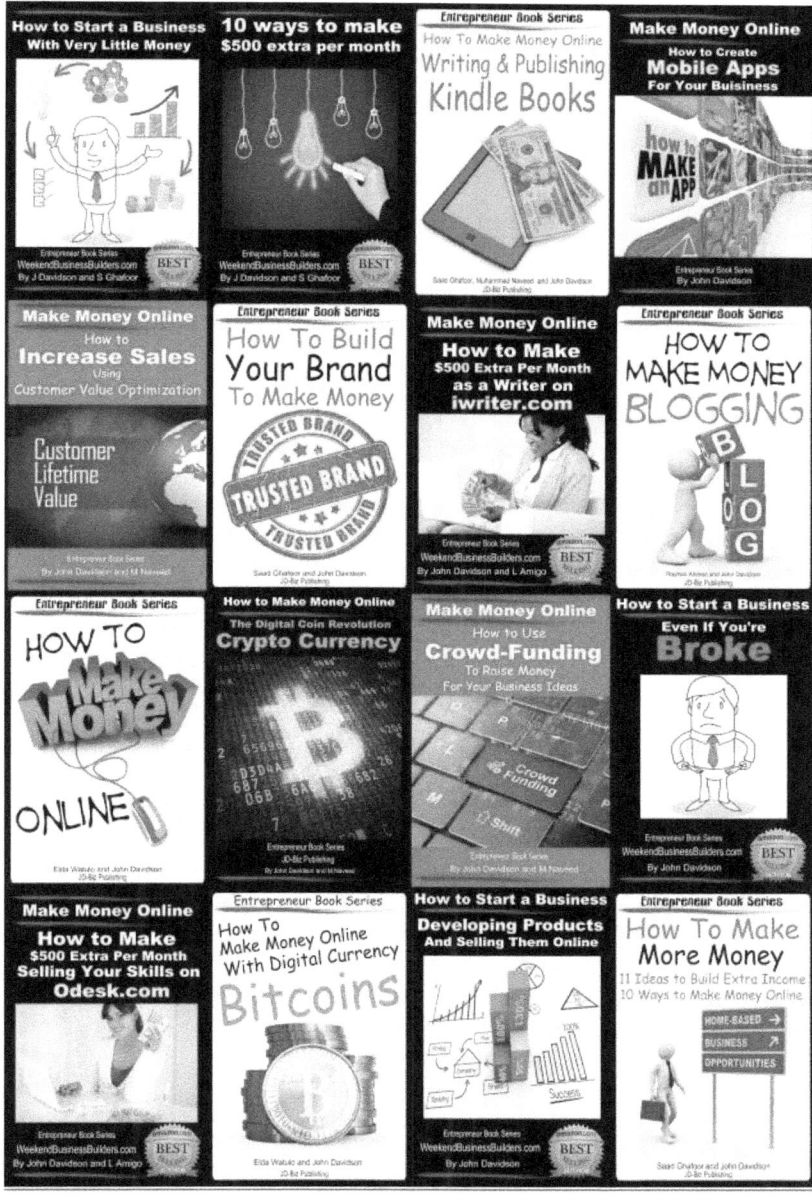

Our books are available at

1. Amazon.com
2. Barnes and Noble
3. Itunes
4. Kobo
5. Smashwords
6. Google Play Books

Publisher

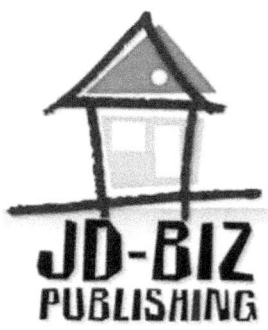

JD-Biz Corp

P O Box 374

Mendon, Utah 84325

http://www.jd-biz.com/

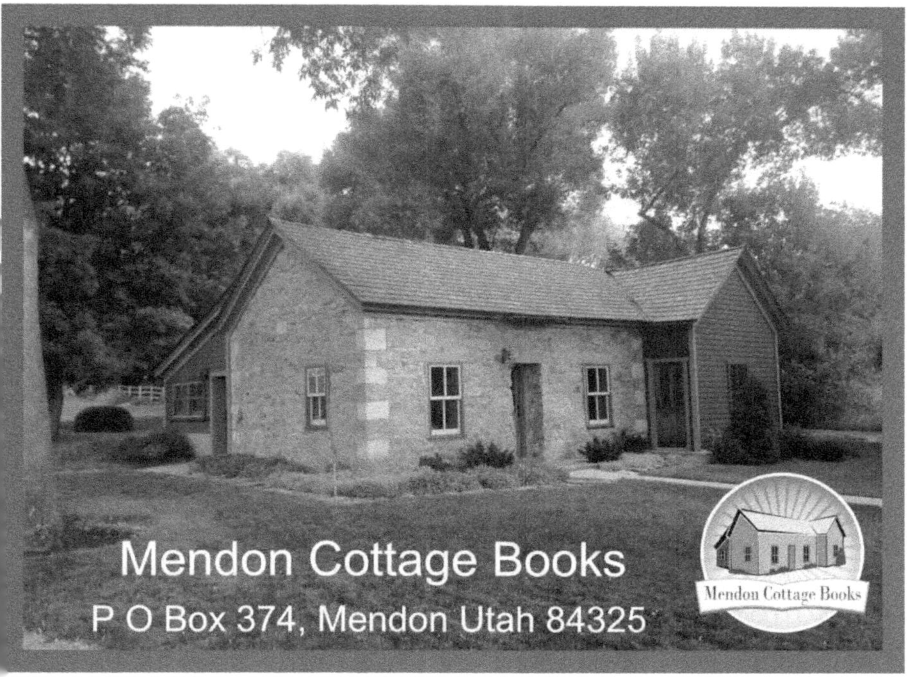

Mendon Cottage Books
P O Box 374, Mendon Utah 84325

www.ingramcontent.com/pod-product-compliance
Lightning Source LLC
Chambersburg PA
CBHW070723180526
45167CB00004B/1593